Atsu Kodjo George KPORVIE

Immunomodulating study of Securidaca longipedunculata (Polygalaceae)

Atsu Kodjo George KPORVIE

Immunomodulating study of Securidaca longipedunculata (Polygalaceae)

Imprint

Any brand names and product names mentioned in this book are subject to trademark, brand or patent protection and are trademarks or registered trademarks of their respective holders. The use of brand names, product names, common names, trade names, product descriptions etc. even without a particular marking in this work is in no way to be construed to mean that such names may be regarded as unrestricted in respect of trademark and brand protection legislation and could thus be used by anyone.

Cover image: www.ingimage.com

This book is a translation from the original published under ISBN 978-620-6-72445-2.

Publisher:
Sciencia Scripts
is a trademark of
Dodo Books Indian Ocean Ltd. and OmniScriptum S.R.L publishing group

120 High Road, East Finchley, London, N2 9ED, United Kingdom
Str. Armeneasca 28/1, office 1, Chisinau MD-2012, Republic of Moldova, Europe
Printed at: see last page
ISBN: 978-620-8-16098-2

Copyright © Atsu Kodjo George KPORVIE
Copyright © 2024 Dodo Books Indian Ocean Ltd. and OmniScriptum S.R.L publishing group

TABLE OF CONTENTS

SUMMARY

Securidaca longipedunculata has long been used to resolve health problems linked to immunological disorders. The immunomodulatory activity associated with Securidaca longipeduncula 's anti-inflammatory effect has yet to be elucidated by scientific research. Qualitative and quantitative assays of the plant's phytochemical compounds were carried out using in vitro tests. The plant's anti-inflammatory activity was assessed using hen egg albumin denaturation inhibition and membrane stabilisation tests. CAT, DPPH and lipoperoxidation inhibition tests were carried out to assess the plant's antioxidant activity in vitro. Immunosuppression was induced in vivo by cyclophosphamide. The immunomodulatory activity of S. longipeduncula was studied by measuring the titer of leucocyte types using the blood cell count (CBC). C-reactive protein was measured to assess the plant's anti-inflammatory activity in vivo. Lactate dehydrogenase titration was used to demonstrate the effect of S. longipeduncula extract on energy balance.

INTRODUCTION

The healthy state of the body, which is a concern for everyone, weighs heavily in the health system of every country in the world without exception. Food processing, new technologies and pollution are leading to a deterioration in the body's homeostasis. The immune system is very important to human health, and all disease is in some way linked to the immune system. At first glance, we might think of any microbial infection (viral such as influenza, Ebola, AIDS, COVID-19; bacterial; fungal or parasitic) that it might be possible to avoid or combat sufficiently with the help of a strengthened immune system, but also of any pathology observed, from allergic disorders and autoimmune diseases to cancers, which are due to a deficient immune system. Good natural and acquired immunity is the key to future health and recovery. It is essential to find a permanent solution to modulate and balance the immune system, reducing the use of chemicals to a strict minimum, as they are responsible for serious undesirable effects **(Beaulieu, 2008)**. The use of natural resources, particularly medicinal plants, is an important alternative to be explored in order to find appropriate solutions to all the ailments and pathologies that threaten humanity. Plant species are very rich in number and diversity. In addition to their role in balancing the ecosystem, plants provide mankind with natural resources that are essential for survival and development. Medicinal plants are a precious heritage for humanity, particularly for the majority of poor communities in developing countries, who depend on them for their primary healthcare and livelihoods **(Salhi et al., 2010)**. Traditional medicine provides relief to over 70% of people in the Third World (**Malaisse, 1992**) and 80% of people in Africa (**Jiofack et al., 2010**). They are therefore a vital resource that can be mobilised for both its health and socio-economic benefits. However, had it not been for the exorbitant cost of modern medicines, the inadequacy of national budgets allocated to health and the inadequacy of health infrastructures, which have forced more than one African government to reconsider the advantages of traditional healthcare systems

(WHO AFR/CR, 2000), the sector would have been largely relegated to the Greek calendar. It is interesting to note that, with the renewed interest in phytotherapy, there is growing concern about its quality, safety and efficacy, given the poor quality of the preparations, the high microbial load characteristic of plants harvested directly from nature, the non-standardised dosages and the limited scientific evidence. It So it's up to all of us to restore the reputation of medicinal plants. Securidaca longipedunculata is one of these plants with health benefits.

S. longipedunculata is one of the species belonging to the "Securidaca" genus, which is widespread in Africa. It is used by traditional practitioners as an antibacterial, antivenin, antiulcer, anticancer and antiheadache agent.... The therapeutic efficacy of this plant is largely due to the presence of secondary metabolites such as flavonoids, xanthones, methyl salicylate, saponins, tannins, anthraquinones, sterols and terpenes Ergotine, sinapic acid, caffeic acid, sucrose, elymoclavin and dihydroelymoclavin in its chemical composition **(Tolo, 2001)**.

Securidaca longipedunculata is a plant with a reputation for being beneficial to a wide range of people in the health field, thanks to the versatility of its potential benefits, including effects associated with modulating the immune system and its anti-inflammatory properties.

This is the context of this study, the general objective of which is to demonstrate the immunomodulatory and anti-inflammatory effects of the hydro-ethanolic extract of S. longipedunculata leaves. This general objective is followed by two specific objectives:

✓ To identify the potential immunomodulatory effect of the hydro-ethanolic extract of S. longipedunculata.
✓ To assess the potential anti-inflammatory effect of the hydro-ethanolic extract of S. longipedunculata.
Thus, our modest work will be divided into two parts: the first deals with a bibliographical summary on immunomodulation, inflammation and plant

material. The second part deals with the experimental study, describing the equipment used, the methods followed and the discussion of the results obtained, and finally a conclusion and research prospects.

LITERATURE REVIEW

Chapter 1: The immune system, inflammation and oxidative stress

I. The immune system

1. The immune system

The immune response can be defined as the integrated action of the mechanisms developed by the body to defend itself against harmful elements in the environment. These mechanisms are brought into play by the body's immune system, i.e. all the molecules in solution in biological fluids and the cells that communicate with each other via mediators and receptors. The immune system therefore has the capacity to recognise agents foreign to the organism, bringing into play two types of reaction: the non-specific, natural or innate response and the specific or adaptive response **(Revillard, 2001 Chatenoud, 2002).**

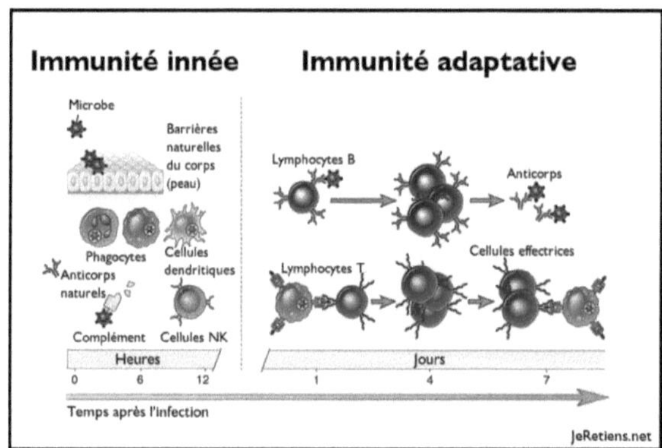

Figure 1: Difference between innate and adaptive immunity **(Mirandole, 2020).**

II. Inflammation

1. Definition of inflammation

The term inflammation comes from the Latin word inflammare, a verb meaning "to set on fire" **(Gruffat, 2021)**. It is the response of living, vascularised tissues to aggression. This aggression involves immunity phenomena **(Laurent, 1988)**. It can be caused by a lack of vascularisation, physical agents (trauma, heat, cold, radiation) or chemical agents (caustics, toxins, venoms), contamination by micro-organisms and dysimmune aggression. It is Inflammation is usually a beneficial process, as its aim is to eliminate the pathogen and repair tissue damage. Sometimes inflammation can be harmful because of the aggressiveness of the pathogen, its persistence, the location of the inflammation, abnormalities in the regulation of the inflammatory process, or quantitative or qualitative abnormalities in the cells involved (**Eldeen et al., 2008**).

2. Acute inflammation

Acute inflammation is the immediate response to an aggressive agent. It lasts for a short time (a few days or weeks), is often sudden in onset and is characterised by intense vasculo-exudative phenomena. Acute inflammation heals spontaneously or with treatment, but can leave sequelae if tissue destruction is significant (**CoPath, 2011**).

3. Chronic inflammation

Chronic inflammation is inflammation that has no tendency to heal spontaneously, and which develops by persisting or worsening over several months or years. There are many diseases with chronic inflammation as a symptom or cause, also known as autoimmune diseases (e.g. ulcerative colitis, certain allergies, rheumatoid arthritis, lupus, chronic fatigue syndrome, sometimes diabetes2) (**Gruffat, 2021**).

4. Clinical signs of inflammation

The clinical signs of inflammation were first described in the 1[er] century AD by a Roman physician named Celsus. He set out the "Quadrilateral of Celsus", describing the symptoms accompanying wound infection: tumor (oedema), rubor (redness), calor (heat) and dolor (pain). These four qualifiers refer to the tissue changes associated with the inflammatory process: dilation of vessels, recruitment of leukocytes and local accumulation of plasma (**Davoust-Nataf, 2021**).

5. Phases of inflammation

The inflammatory reaction is a dynamic process comprising several successive phases: the vasculo-exudative phase, the cellular reaction, detersion and the final phase of repair and healing.

5.1. Vasculo-exudative or vasculo-sanguinous phase or initiation

Clinically, it is characterised by the four classic cardinal signs of acute inflammation: redness, heat, swelling and pain. During this phase, three phenomena follow one another: active congestion, inflammatory oedema and leukocyte diapedesis (**Rousselet et al., 2005**).

5.1.1. Active congestion

This involves arteriolar and then capillary vasodilatation in the affected area. Locally, this results in an increase in blood supply and a slowdown in circulatory flow. Congestion is triggered rapidly by a nervous mechanism (vasomotor nerves) and the action of chemical mediators (**CoPath, 2011**).

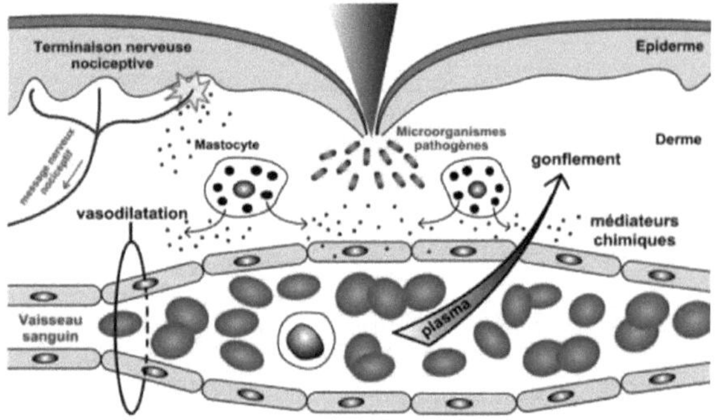

Figure 5: Progression of the vasculo-exudative phase (**Prin et al.,2009**).

5.1.2. Inflammatory oedema

It is caused by the infiltration of connective tissue, serous cavities, joint cavities and pulmonary alveoli by a liquid called exudate, consisting of water and blood proteins: albumin, coagulation factors, fibrinogen, enzymes and immunoglobulins. Inflammatory oedema results from an increase in hydrostatic pressure due to vasodilatation and, above all, an increase in the permeability of the walls of the small vessels under the effect of chemical mediators, including histamine (**Aouissa, 2002**).

The role of this inflammatory stage is to provide local chemical mediators and means of defence (immunoglobulins, coagulation factors, complement factors); to dilute the toxins accumulated in the lesion; to limit the inflammatory focus with a fibrin barrier (derived from plasma fibrinogen) to prevent the spread of infectious micro-organisms; to slow down the circulatory flow by haemoconcentration to encourage the next stage: leukocyte diapedesis (**CoPath, 2011**).

5.1.3. Leukocyte diapedesis

Leukocyte diapedesis corresponds to the migration of leukocytes outside the microcirculation and their accumulation in the lesion site. It is the passage of leukocytes through the wall of a dilated capillary. It initially involves the polymorphonuclear cells (during the first 6 to 24 hours), then a monocytes and lymphocytes a little later (in 24 to 48 hours) (**CoPath, 2011**).

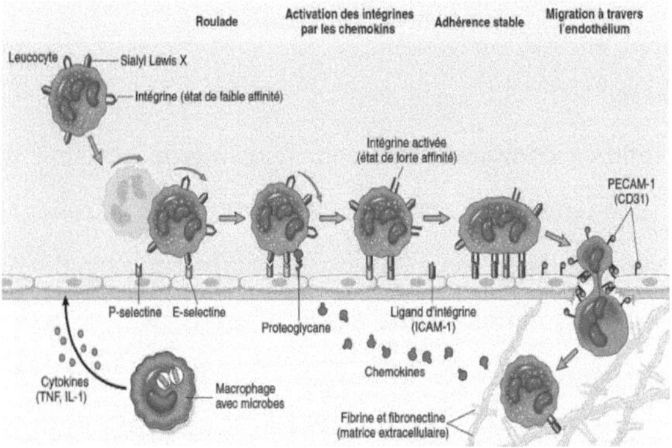

Figure 6: Leukocyte diapedesis.

The leukocytes undergo a rolling process, are then activated and adhere to the endothelium, and finally cross the endothelium and move towards the site of the inflammatory reaction along a chemoattractant gradient. Several molecules play an important role in this multi-step process: selectins for rolling, chemokines for leukocyte and integrin activation (transition to a high-affinity state), integrins for stable adhesion to the endothelium, and CD-31 (PECAM1) for migration through the vascular wall (**Mury, 2018**).

5.2. The cell phase

This corresponds to the formation of the inflammatory granuloma. The inflammatory site rapidly becomes enriched with cells from the blood and local connective tissue. Infiltrated cells include mast cells, macrophages, neutrophils and lymphocytes. These cells aggregate due to the high production of chemoattractant factors (**Rousselet et al., 2005**).

5.3. Detersion

It gradually follows the vasculo-exudative phase, and is contemporary with the cellular phase. Detersion can be compared to cleaning the lesion site: it involves eliminating necrotic tissue from the initial attack or from the inflammatory process itself, pathogens and exudate. Detersion is a necessary preparation for the final phase of repair and healing. If detersion is incomplete, acute inflammation will develop into chronic inflammation.

5.4. Repair phase

Tissue repair follows complete detersion. It results in scarring if the damaged tissue cannot regenerate (e.g. neurons or myocardial muscle cells) or when tissue destruction has been very extensive and/or prolonged. The repair may result in complete restoration of the tissue: there is then no trace of the initial attack and the inflammation that followed. This highly favourable outcome is observed in the case of limited, brief, relatively non-destructive attacks on tissue capable of cellular regeneration (**Zerbato, 2010**).

The stages of tissue repair are the fleshy bud and healing: the fleshy bud and healing.

6. Anti-inflammatory drugs

Anti-inflammatories (AI) are symptomatic drugs that do not act on the cause of inflammation. They are indicated when inflammation, a normal process of defence against aggression, becomes bothersome, particularly because of the pain it causes. IAs also have an analgesic and antipyretic action (**Thomas, 2017**).

CEWs fall into two categories:

– Non-steroidal anti-inflammatory drugs (NSAIDs)

– Corticosteroids, i.e. steroidal anti-inflammatory drugs.

6.1.Non-steroidal anti-inflammatory drugs (NSAIDs)

In addition to their anti-inflammatory properties, they also have analgesic and antipyretic properties (**Cohen, 1981**). These three properties are essentially due to their common mechanism of action: inhibition of prostaglandin biosynthesis via cyclooxygenase isoenzymes (COX-1 and COX-2) (**Manciaux, 1993**). The COX-1 and COX-2 enzymes catalyse the conversion of arachidonic acid into prostaglandin H2, an intermediate metabolite in the formation of prostaglandins. The activity of the various prostaglandins in a given tissue depends on the expression of specific receptors and enzymes (prostaglandin synthases) involved in their biosynthesis. Classical NSAIDs inhibit the activity of COX-1 and COX-2, while that coxibs such as celecoxib, parecoxib and etoricoxib selectively inhibit the COX-2 enzyme (**Meunier, 2018**; **Juneau, 2017**). NSAIDs therefore lead to a reduction in prostaglandin biosynthesis and associated biological activities (**Vane, 1971**). COX-1 is constitutively expressed in most tissues, whereas COX-2 is expressed in only a few tissues. COX-2 expression can be induced in response to inflammatory stimuli and it is through this mechanism that prostaglandin levels increase in sites of inflammation (e.g. joints). Conventional NSAIDs inhibit all biological activities for this, whereas coxibs are active in certain tissues only because of their selectivity for COX-2 (**Juneau,**

2017).

Depending on the inhibitory mechanism, we have :

✓ Irreversible inhibitors: of all the NSAIDs, only ASPIRIN has the capacity to irreversibly inactivate COX-1 and COX-2, by acetylation of the enzymatic active site.

✓ Reversible competitive inhibitors: they form a rapidly dissociable complex with COX (examples: IBUPROFEN, MEFENAMIC ACID, PIROXICAM).

✓ Time-dependent reversible inhibitors: some NSAIDs, such as INDOMETACIN, form a slowly dissociable complex with the enzyme (ionic interactions with the enzyme site) (**Nuhrich, 2015**).

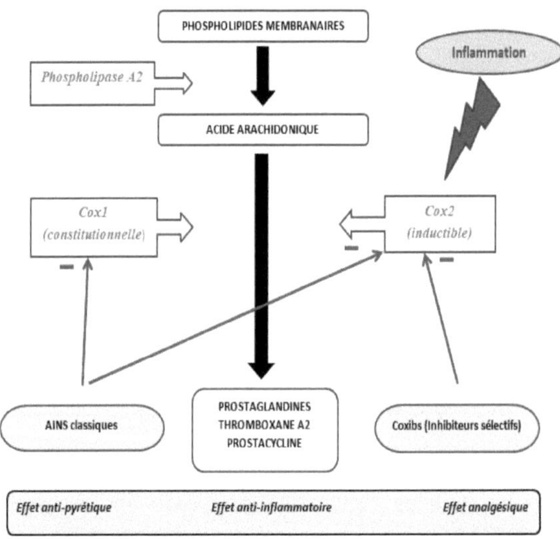

Figure 7: Mechanism of action of NSAIDs.

6.2. Steroidal anti-inflammatories

Steroidal anti-inflammatories (SIAs) or glucocorticoids are more potent than NSAIDs (**Gruffat, 2021**). They are derivatives of natural hormones secreted by the adrenal cortex or hemi-synthesised from animal or plant extracts (**Coyen, 1981**).

They are derived from cholesterol and their production is stimulated by ACTH.

The reference endogenous glucocorticoid is cortisol. It is produced by cells in the fascicular zone of the adrenal cortex.

Cortisol, also known as hydrocortisone, not only has anti-inflammatory properties but also mineralocorticoid properties (anti-diuretic, anti-natriuretic and kaliuretic). Synthetic glucocorticoids are medicines derived from the natural hormone cortisol, and were developed to maximise glucocorticoid effects and minimise mineralocorticoid effects. They include three classes of drugs:

✓ Corticosteroids in combination: Celestamine, Ciloxadex.

✓ Non-associated glucocorticoids: Altim, Betamethasone, Betnesol, Celestene, Cortancyl, Decadron, Dectancyl, Dexamethasone, Diprostene, Hexatrione, Hydrocortancyl, Medrol, Methylprednisolone, Neodex, Neofordex, Prednisolone.

✓ Non-associated mineralocorticoids: Adixon, Florinef, Flucortac (**CNPM, 2018**).

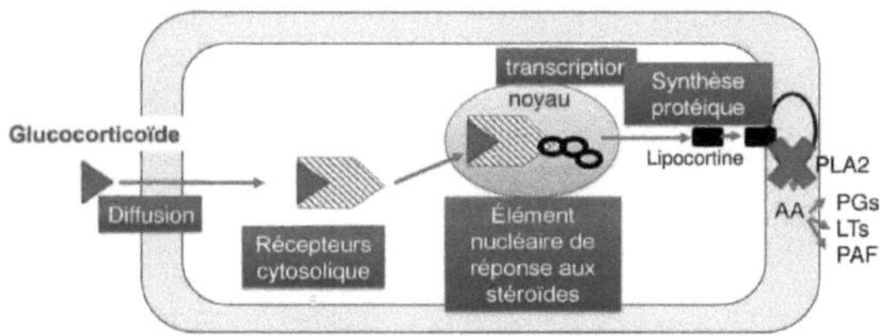

Figure 8: Genomic effect of corticosteroids (**Ferran, 2013**)

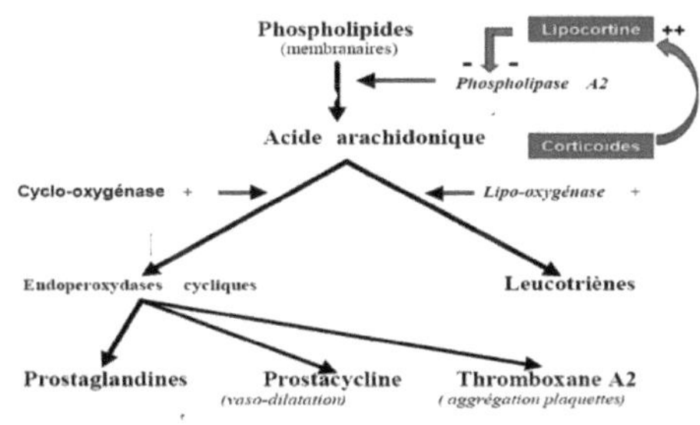

Figure 9: Effect of corticoids on the inflammation process (Rasamindrakotroka, 2013)

III. Oxidative stress

1. Definition

Oxidative stress is recognised as a n alteration in redox homeostasis **(Favier, 2003)**, leading to potential cell damage. During a Oxidative stress: reactive oxygen species that are not "detoxified" by the antioxidant system attack and damage macromolecules, particularly lipids, proteins and DNA **(Koechlin-Ramonatxo, 2006)**.

2. Free radicals

A free radical is a chemical entity (atom, molecule, fragment of a molecule) that has one or more unpaired or single electrons in its external orbitals. It reacts spontaneously with other atoms or molecules to form a new radical, triggering a chain reaction **(Favier, 2003; Gardés et al., 2003)**.

3. Oxygen Reactive Species

Among the enzymatic reactions, several are considered to be the main source of reactive oxygen species (ROS), including : NADPH oxidase, lipoxygenase, xanthine oxidase (enzyme in the liver). The mitochondrion is fundamental to the functioning of the cell, as it is in this organelle that cellular respiration takes place. The consumption of oxygen and the various electron transfer reactions (energy) produce reactive oxygen species. Metal ions present in the body, e.g. iron and copper, can cooperate with less reactive species to produce hydroxyl radicals **(Poprac et al., 2017)**.

ROS are also generated under the effect of environmental stresses such as pollution, alcohol consumption or certain drugs, prolonged exposure to sunlight, intense exertion as well as smoking. **(Kalam et al., 2015)**.

The major ROS of physiological significance are superoxide anion, hydroxyl radical and hydrogen peroxide **(Gardès et al., 2003)**.

4. Antioxidants

The term "antioxidant" covers a range of different activities in which several molecular species slow down or prevent the oxidation of biological substrates **(Athamena et al., 2010)**.

4.1. Primary antioxidants

They are produced by our bodies, and include specific factors such as glutathione, alpha-lipoic acid and uric acid, as well as enzymes (catalase, glutathione reductase, superoxide dismutase) which require the presence of minerals from food to be activated: iron, zinc, copper and selenium **(Causse, 1994)**.

4.2 Secondary antioxidants

These are exogenous molecules that can act as antioxidants in vivo, including vitamin E, ascorbic acid, βcarotene, flavonoids and phenolic compounds.

4.3. Antioxidants of plant origin

The body uses numerous antioxidant strategies, including those provided by food, such as vitamin E, vitamin C, carotenoids, flavonoids and polyphenols.

PLANT MATERIAL

I. Herbal medicine

The word phytotherapy comes from two Greek words, phyton: plant and therapeuein: to heal, which essentially mean "to heal with plants". It is an age-old practice based on empirical knowledge that has been passed down and enriched over countless generations **(Sadok, 2008)**.

II. Medicinal plant

A medicinal plant is a plant used for its therapeutic properties. This means that at least one of its parts (leaves, bulbs, roots, seeds, fruits, flowers) can be used to cure **(Petrovska, 2012)** or prevent a disease.

They have been used by man since at least 7,000 BC and form the basis of phytotherapy. Their effectiveness is based on their compounds, which are very numerous and varied depending on the species, and which are all different active ingredients **(Vidal, 2010)**.

III. Securidaca longipedunculata monograph

The generic name **Securidaca longipedunculata** comes from the Latin :

- **Securis**, meaning axe of meaning

- **longipedunculata**, meaning long stalk **(Ndou, 2010)**.

Common names

Table 4: Vernacular names for S. longepelunculata in various African countries.

Pays	Langues locales	courantes	Noms de *Securidaca longipedunculata*
Burkina Faso	Mooré		Palgu, Pélga
	Dioula		Djoro; Djoto
Cote d'Ivoire	Lobi		Samuele
	Malinké		Diulo, Ndjuru
Gambie	Malinké		Juto, Djuto
	Fula		Alali
Ghana	Akan		Ofodo, Kyrito
Guinée	Malinké		Diodo,
Conakry	Fula		Diantu
Mali	Bambara		Djoro, Dioro
	Dogon		Toroe
	Peulh		Iguili,
Niger	Hausa		Warnagunguna
	Fula		Adali
	Djerma		Hasukore
Nigéria	Hausa		Sanya
	Fula		Adali
	Yoruba		Ipeta
Sénégal	Diola		Fu Daray
	Wolof		Fuf
Sierra Leone	Malinké		Juto, Jodoo (OOAS, 2013)
Tanzanie	Iringa		M'yangabako (Joseph *et al.*, 2006)
Togo	Ouatchi		Etritu
	Ewé		Kpeta, Etritu, Metritu
	Kotokoli		fose

Herbarium specimen number **(WAHO, 2013)** :

Ghana: 2799Mali: 0058Togo: TOGO06917

IV. Botanical data

1. Classification

Table 5: Position of the plant in systematics **(Mathias, 1982)**

Règne	Végétal
Embranchement	Spermaphyte
Sous embranchement	Angiosperme
Classe	Dicotylédone
Sous classe	Dialypétale
Série	Disciflore
Sous série	Diplostemone
Ordre	Sapindale
Famille	Polygalaceae
Genre	*Securidaca*
Espèce	*longipedunculata*

2. Description of the plant

It is an upright shrub, 3 to 4 m high, with slender, drooping branches that are more or less pubescent. The stem is usually pubescent at first, then becomes hairless; the bark is smooth, light yellow with a green film and pale yellow wood. The leaves are alternate, oblong, linear or elliptical, rounded at the apex, slightly pubescent or hairless on both sides, 2 to 5 cm long, with a short pubescent petiole 2 to 3 mm long. The papilionaceous flowers are pink or purple. They appear mainly in the dry season during leaf-thinning, in the form of short clusters. They are highly ornamental and fragrant, with five sepals, two of which are toothed, and petaloids, a large petal and two lateral petals. The fruits are samaras up to 4 to 5 cm long with a curved membranous wing about 1.5 to 2 cm wide. The seeds are generally rough, which makes growing the plant difficult, although some authors recommend that they should be carefully soaked and planted in isolated sandy soil. The roots are tortuous, rough and light yellow in colour. They are very thick, and give off a characteristic odour like pyrole oil **(Tolo, 2001)**.

V. Uses of S. longipedunculata in traditional African medicine

Securidaca longipedunculata is a plant that is widely used in tropical Africa to treat sickle cell anaemia, aches and pains, amoebiasis, intestinal worms, malaria and to protect animals, This is why the plant is called "arbuste à serpent" in French and "Fuf" in Wolof, which is an onomatopoeia reminiscent of a snake hissing **(Kerharo and Adam, 1974)**. The plant is said to be an intra-vaginal poison in South Africa, where female suicides are frequently committed by inserting it into the vagina.

VI. Phytochemical data

Chemists at the Imperial Institute in London have reported the presence of methyl salicylate and saponin in the roots. Moers demonstrated in 1966 that S. longipedunculata contained the same sapogenin, senegenin, found in Polygala senega **(Tolo, 2001)**. Sugars (glucose, rhamnose, galactose and arabinose) and aglycones from Polygala senega such as presenegine, senegenine, securunine, senegenic acid and dihydrochlorosenegenine have been isolated from S. longipedunculata **(Declaude, 1971)**. Elymoclavin and dihydroelymoclavin are also present in the roots **(Costa et al., 1992)**. The leaves of S. longipedunculata contained saponins, tannins, anthraquinones, sterols and terpenes, but no flavonoids **(Odebiyi, 1978)**.

VII. Pharmacological data

Numerous studies have been carried out on Securidaca longipedunculata Fresen: Aqueous and choroform extracts of roots have shown anti-bacterial activity against many germs, including Bacilus substilis and Escherichia coli, Klebsilla pneumoniae, Proteus vulgaris, Pseudomonas aeroginosa, Salmonella gallinarium, Staphylococus albus and Staphylococus aureus **(Almagboul et al., 1985; Joseph et al., 2006)**.

Aqueous ethanol, methanol and acetone extracts of the roots and/or leaves have shown specific antimicrobial activity against Escherichia coli, Plasmodium, Shigella sp. and Salmonella typhus, as well as anti-diarrhoeal activity **(Junaid, 2008)**; anti-staphylococcal activity **(Namadina et al, 2020; Tauheed, 2017; Tiksa, 2019)**; anti-plasmodial and anticonvulsant **(Bah et al., 2007)**; anti-HIV **(Mahmood et al., 1993. Beuscher et al., 1994)**.

The 60% methanolic extract of Securidaca longipedunculata (Fresen.) root bark inhibited frog rectus abdominis muscle contractions induced by acetycholine, arbachol or nicotine (0.1-10 mg/ml) in a dose-dependent manner **(Ojewole, 2000)**. Xanthones isolated from roots have been shown to stimulate the erectile function of the cavernous muscle in men suffering from erectile dysfunction **(Meyer et al., 2008)**.

Securidaca longipedunculata root extract produced a significant (P < 0.05) dose-dependent alteration in serum enzymes and urea.

Wannang et al (2006) revealed the plant's anti-venomous properties.

The plant's analgesic, anti-inflammatory, hypoglycaemic and depressant activities have been demonstrated using the roots and leaves **(Tolo, 2001; Okoli, 2006; Adebiyi, 2006; Ojewode, 2008; Elufioye, 2014, Silla, 2018**; **Kola et al, 2022)**.

Studies have shown that methanol, ethyl acetate and hexane extracts of S. longipedunculata leaves are potent gastro-protective and anti-ulcer agents **(Kayode, 2015)**.

Studies carried out in Ghana have shown that the roots provide strong pesticidal activity **(Jayasekara et al., 2005; Buxton et al., 2014)**.

VIII.   Toxicological data

The aqueous extract of Securidaca longipedunculata root bark was found to have an LD50 value of 771 mg/kg body weight when administered orally to rats, indicating that root bark is mildly toxic to laboratory animals **(Auwal et al., 2012)**.

MATERIALS AND METHODS

I. Study framework

Our study was carried out in the physiopathology-bioactive substances and safety research unit of the Faculty of Science at the University of Lomé.

II. Study materials

1. Plant material

It consists of Securidaca longipedunculata leaves harvested in June 2022 in LODZI, a village about 15 km west of the town of ANIÉ. The plant was identified and deposited under number TOGO06917 in the herbarium of the Faculty of Science at the University of Lomé.

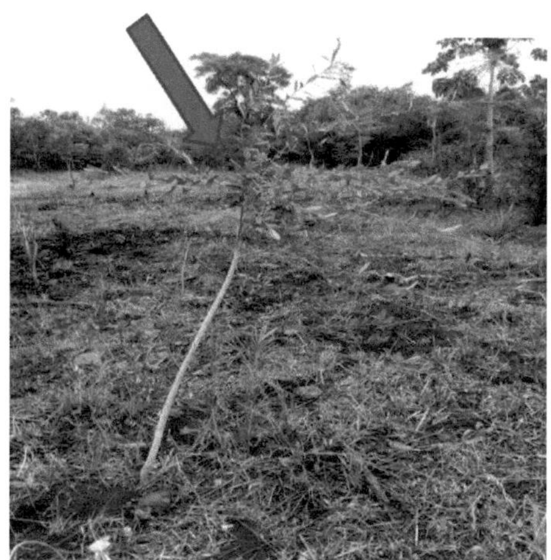

Photo 1: Twigs of S. longipedunculata

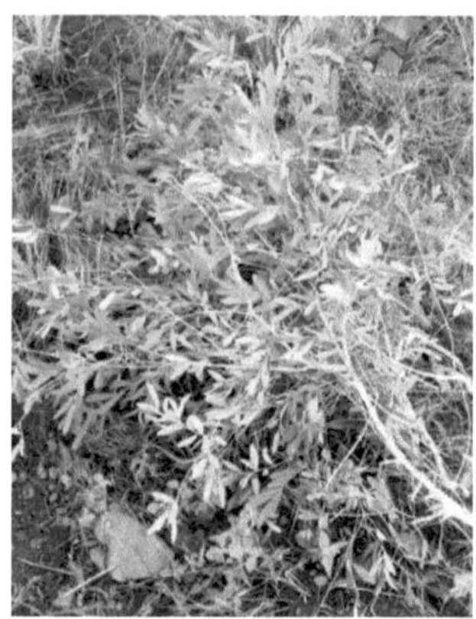

Photo 2: Young plant of S. longipedunculata (Source: photographs, KPORVIE Atsu, 30 June 2022).

2. Animal material

Sprague-dawley rats (male and female) were used in this study. They were selected according to their age (8 to 10 weeks) and weight (150 to 180g). The animals were bred at the Animal Physiology Department of the University of Lomé. The experimental animals were kept in a room at room temperature, $27\pm2°C$ and a 12H/12H light/dark cycle, with free access to drinking water and food. All tests using rats, blood and eggs were carried out with the approval of the Ethics Committee of the Department of Animal Physiology at the University of Lomé, a branch of the Ethics Committee for the control and supervision of animal experiments and the use of blood, Ref n° 006/2020 / BC-BPA / FDS-UL.

3. Chemicals used

Cyclophosphamide, distilled water, ethanol, rutin, ferric chloride, NaOH, bisaublimated iodine, potassium iodide, basic bismuth nitrate, acetic acid, sulphuric acid, ether, levamisole.

4. Other equipment

Dry tubes, micropipettes, pipettes, syringes, beakers, stopwatch, notebook, pen, cotton wool, cages, measuring cylinders, spectrophotometer, thermostable bath, automats, general-purpose laboratory equipment.

III. Methods

1. Preparing plant material

The leaves of S. longipedunculata were harvested and dried at laboratory temperature, protected from light and humidity. After drying, they were collected and stored in a dry place.

2. Hydroethanol extract

Hydroethanol extraction is based on water and ethanol. To do this, 500g of S. longipedunculata leaf powder was macerated for 72h in the absence of air, in 5L of a mixture of water and ethanol of equal volume (50/50, v/v). The preparation was filtered twice using cotton wool and then Whatman No. 1 paper. The extracts were evaporated to dryness using a rotavapor. The extracts obtained were weighed and stored in tubes at 4°C protected from light until use. The extraction yield was determined by the following formula:

$$Rendement = \frac{Masse\ du\ résidu\ sec\ de\ l'extrait\ évaporé}{Masse\ de\ la\ poudre\ la\ matière\ végétale\ sèche} X\ 100$$

2.1 Preliminary phytochemical screening of S. longipedunculata

The hydroethanol extract of S. longipedunculata was dissolved in distilled water and then filtered. The filtrate was used to test for certain chemical compounds using the method of **Kpoyizoun et al. (2020)** as shown in **Table 6**.

Table 6: Protocol for identifying the main chemical groups

Groupes chimiques	Réactifs	Extrait de *S. longipedunculata*
Flavonoïdes	Chlorure ferrique 1%	Coloration jaune orangé
	NaOH 1/10	Coloration verdâtre
Tannins	Chlorure ferrique 1%	Coloration bleu-noire
Saponosides	Test de mousse	Mousse persistante pendant 15 min
Alcaloïdes	Bouchardart (iode bisaublimé + iodure de potassium + eau)	Précipité brun
	Dragendorf (Nitrate basique de Bismuth + acide acétique + eau)	Précipité orangé
	Mayer (iode + iodure de potassium + eau)	Précipité blanc ou blanc jaunâtre
Glucides	Réactif de Molish (α-naphtol) + H_2SO_4	Anneau rouge

3.2. Quantitative determination of phytochemical compounds

3.2.1. Determination of total flavonoids

Flavonoids were assayed by the calorimetric method using aluminium chloride. This method is based on the properties of flavonoids to form aluminium chelates with aluminium chloride **(Kola et al., 2022)**. To 2mL of extract (1mg/mL) or rutin (1mg/mL), 2mL of aluminium chloride (2%) and 6mL of sodium acetate (50 mg/mL) were added. The blank was made with 2ml ethanol in place of the sample. The OD was read at 440nm after 30 minutes. The total flavonoid content of the S. longipedunculata extract was determined from the linear regression equation of the calibration range

established with rutin (5µg/mL, 25µg/mL, 50 µg/mL, 100 µg/mL, 200 µg/mL) and expressed in µg rutin equivalent per milligram of dry extract (µg EQ/mg extract). Rutin is taken as the reference. The tests were repeated three times.

3.2.2. Determination of phenols and tannins

The total phenol content of the extract is determined by the calorimetric method using the Folin-Ciocalteu reagent **(Dosseh et al., 2014)** after fixation of the tannins by PVPP (polyvinylpolypyrrolidone). This method involves two steps:

Step 1: 500 µL of the extract (stock solution at 1mg/mL) was transferred to tubes containing 10 mg of PVPP and methanol. The resulting mixture was incubated on ice for 30 minutes. After centrifugation, 200 µL of the supernatant was transferred to dry tubes for assay with Folin-Ciocalteu reagent. The blank was prepared with 1mL of methanol in place of the extract.

Step 2: To 200 µL of the extract solution (stock solution at 1mg/mL) or 200 µL of the gallic acid solutions (50, 25, 12.5, 6.25 and 0 µg/mL) or 200 µL of the solution obtained in step 1 (extract + PVPP), 200 µL of 10% Folin-Ciocalteu reagent (10-fold diluted in distilled water) was added. After 10min incubation at room temperature, 750µL of sodium carbonate ($Na_2 CO_3$) (60g/L) was added. The optical density (OD) was read on a spectrometer at 725nm against a blank. The amount of total phenol is expressed in terms of mg gallic acid equivalent/g extract. The total amount of tannin was calculated using the following formula:

3.3. In vitro anti-inflammatory test

3.3.1. Egg albumin denaturation inhibition test

DOT= DO tannins; DOE= DO extract; DOE+PVPP= DO extract + PVPP

The test was performed according to the method of **Saleem et al (2020)**. The reaction mixture (5ml) consisted of 0.2ml egg albumin from fresh hen egg, 2.8ml PBS (Ph 6.4) and 2ml extract or reference drug (Diclofenac sodium) at different concentrations (500, 250, 125 62.5 and 0µg/ml). The control and test samples were incubated at 37°C for 25 minutes and then at 70°C for 5 minutes. After cooling to 37°C, the optical density of each sample was measured at 660 nm and the percentage inhibition of protein denaturation, which determines anti-inflammatory activity, was calculated using the formula :

$$Activité\ anti - inflammatoire\ (\%) = \left(1 - \frac{At}{Ac}\right) X\ 100$$

Ac = absorbance of the negative control and At = absorbance of the test performed

3.3.2. Membrane stabilisation test

The method used was that of **Javed et al (2020)**. The rats were first anaesthetised with ether and then 5 ml of blood was drawn from the retro-orbital sinus into heparin tubes. The blood was centrifuged at 1500 rpm for 10 minutes to separate the erythrocytes from the plasma and buffy coat. The erythrocytes were then washed three times with the same normal saline solution. The resulting erythrocyte pellet was then suspended in 10 volumes of normal saline.

3.3.2.1. Haemolysis induced by hypotonic solution

Reference drug (aspirin) at different concentrations (25- 200µg/ml) or 1ml S. longipedunculata extract and 2ml hyposaline solution (0.36%) were added to 1ml erythrocyte suspension. After 30 minutes incubation at 37°C, the mixtures were centrifuged at 3000 rpm for 15 minutes and then the optical density was read at 560 nm. All measurements were repeated 3 times. The percentage of membrane stabilisation, which reflects the anti-inflammatory activity, was determined using the following formula:

$$Activité\ anti - inflammatoire\ (\%) = \left(1 - \frac{At}{Ac}\right) X\ 100$$

Ac = absorbance of the negative control and At = absorbance of the test performed

3.3.2.2. Heat-induced haemolysis

To 1ml of the erythrocyte suspension was added 1ml of extract or reference drug (aspirin or diclofenac) at different concentrations (25-200µg/ml). The mixture was then incubated at 56°C in a water bath for 30 minutes. After cooling, the solutions were centrifuged at 2,500 rpm and the absorbance of the supernatant was read at 560nm. The percentage inhibition is calculated using the following formula.

3.4. Antioxidant activity of S. longipedunculata in vitro

3.4.1. Total antioxidant capacity (phosphomolybdenum assay)

The test is based on the reduction of molybdenum Mo (VI) present in the form of molybdate ions MoO_4^{2-} to molybdenum Mo (V) MoO^{2+} in the presence of the extract or an antioxidant agent. This reduction results in the formation of a greenish complex (phosphate/Mo(V)) at an acid pH **(Prieto et al., 1999)**. The increase in colour of the molybdenum (VI) complex is measured in the presence of antioxidant.

The method involves introducing 1000 µg/ml of S. longipedunculata extract into a tube mixed with 3ml of a reagent consisting of $H_2 SO_4$ (0.6 M), $Na_2 PO_4$ (28 mM) and ammonium molybdate (4 mM). The tube was then tightly closed and incubated at 95°C for 90 minutes. After cooling, absorbance was measured at 695 nm. The control consists of 100µl of ethanol mixed with 1000 µl of the reagent mentioned above. The samples and controls were incubated under the same conditions

3.4.2. Evaluation of anti-free radical activity using the DPPH (2,2-diphenyl-1-picrylhydrzyl

The DPPH (diphenylpicrylhydrazyl) method is based on the reduction of the stable radical species DPPH- in the presence of a hydrogen-donating antioxidant (AH), resulting in the formation of a non-radical form, DPPH-H (diphenyl picrylhydrazine). In the presence of free radical scavengers, the violet-coloured DPPH- is reduced to the yellow-coloured DPPH.H. The reduction of the DPPH free radical can be monitored by UV visible spectrometry, by measuring the decrease in absorbance at 517 nm **(Athamena et al., 2010)**.

Procedure :

To a volume of 3ml of different (3.125 µg/ml to 100 µg/ml) extract or standard solution of ascorbic acid is added 1ml of 0.1mM of the freshly prepared ethanolic solution of DPPH. After incubation in the dark for 30 min at room temperature, absorbance readings were taken at 517 nm using a spectrophotometer.The percentage of inhibition is calculated using the following formula:

$$I\,(\%) = \left(1 - \frac{At}{Ac}\right) X\ 100$$

3.4.3. Inhibition of lipoperoxidation induced by FeCl2-ascorbic acid on bone marrow homogenate.

> **Determination of MDA (malondialdehyde)**

The anti-lipid peroxidation effect of the extract was studied using the method of **Kpemissi et al. (2019b).** Bone marrow tissue was rapidly removed from sacrificed rats. A 2g piece of bone marrow was cut and homogenised with10 mL of 150 mM Tris HCl KCl buffer (PH 7.4). The reaction mixture consisted of 500 Ul organ homogenate, 200 µL 150 mM KCl Tris HCl buffer (PH 7.4), 100 µL of 0.1 mM ascorbic acid, 100 µL of 4 mM $FeCl_2$ and 100 µL of various concentrations of securidaca longipedunculata extract or standard. This mixture was incubated at 37°C for 1 hour in stoppered tubes. MDA concentration was estimated as described previously **(Kpemissi et al., 2019b).** MDA levels as a marker of lipid peroxidation were analysed by a calorimetric assay based on the reaction of MDA with a chromogenic reagent to give a stable chromophore with a maximum absorbance at 586 nm. Briefly, 650 µL of 10.3 Mm 1-methyl-2-phenyl-indole in acetonitrile diluted with 32 mM methanol (3:1) was added to 250 u µL of each sample and the mixture vortexed. After adding 150 µL of 37% (v/v) HCl, the samples were tightly capped and incubated at 45°C for one hour. The samples were then cooled, centrifuged at 4000rpm for 10min and the absorbance measured spectrometrically at 586nm. A standard curve of 1,1,3,3-

tetra-methoxypropane was also performed for the quantification of MDA.

➤ Determination of total protein in bone marrow tissue

The protein content of the experimental samples was measured by the Bradford method using crystalline bovine serum albumin (BSA) as a standard **(Kpemissi et al., 2019b).** To 15 µL of homogenate or BSA at different concentrations, 750 µL of Bradford reagent was added. The absorbance was read 5 minutes later at 595 nm.

3. Immunomodulatory and anti-inflammatory activity in vivo

4.1. Distribution of animals and design

They were given no food before the treatment. They were divided into 5 groups of 5 rats, each treated or not.

Table 7: Breakdown of animals and design for in vivo tests

Control Group (G. Control	Cyclo Group (G. Cyclo)	Extracted group 200 + Cyclo (G. Extract 200)	400+ extracted group Cyclo (G. Extract 400)	Levamisole + Cyclo group (G. Levamisole)
Distilled water 10mg/kg (d0- d13) +	Distilled water (d0- d13) +	Extract 200mg/kg (d0- d13) +	Extract 400mg/kg (d0- d13) + Cyclo	Levamisole 30mg/kg (d0- d13)
1ml/Kg 0.9% NaCl (d11-d13)	Cyclo 30mg/kg (d11-d13)	Cyclo 30mg/kg (d11-d13)	30mg/kg (d11- d13)	+ Cyclo 30mg/kg (j11-j13)

4.2. Sampling

After the treatment period, the animals were sacrificed, the blood collected in dry tubes and tubes containing EDTA. The blood sample was centrifuged at 3500 t.p.m for 10 min. The supernatant (serum) is used for the determination of biochemical and enzymatic parameters. The whole blood from the EDTA tubes is used for counting the blood count.

4.3. Blood count (CBC)

Blood counts were carried out using an automated system based on flow cytometry.

Principle: Cells suspended in a liquid flow pass one by one through a laser beam. The physical scattering of the light emitted by the light source depends on the cell size and granularity (granule content, more or less segmented structure of the nucleus). Scattering in the direction of the light source (forward scatter, FSC) provides information on size, while scattering at 90°C (side scatter, SSC) provides information on granularity or structure. An electronic system converts the optical signals (photons) into electronic signals. The signals are collected by photomultipliers, amplified, digitised and stored in a computer. A computer system displays the signals.

4.4. Determination of CRP (C-Reactive Protein) or Pantraxin 1.

CRP is a protein belonging to the pentraxin family. It plays a role in the immune response, binding to immunoglobulin G and activating the complement system, mobilising and activating leukocytes and stimulating phagocytosis. It is mainly found in blood serum. It is an early, sensitive and specific marker of the inflammatory reaction, and is proportional to its intensity **(Gloaguen, 2007).**

CRP was measured in rat serum using an automated system.

4.5. Assessment of lactate dehydrogenase (LDH) enzyme activity

Lactate dehydrogenase (LDH) is a ubiquitous intracellular enzyme. The highest concentrations of LDH are found in the liver, heart, kidneys, skeletal muscle and erythrocytes. It catalyses the reversible conversion of pyruvate to lactate in the presence of NAD+/NADH. The following reaction :

LDH was also measured in rat serum using an automated system.

IV. Data analysis

The results were presented as the mean plus or minus the standard error of the mean (SEM). They were processed using Graph Pad Prism 8.0.1 software, which is also used to construct histograms. Tukey's multiple comparison test was used to compare the means of the data. The differences between the results were considered significant at the 5% threshold (p value < 0.05).

RESULTS

I. Yield of S. longipedunculata extract

Table 8: Extract yield

Matériel végétal	Aspect	Couleur	Rendement (%)
Feuilles de *longipedunculata*	*S.* Visqueux	Marron	15.05

II. Phytochemical screening

1. Qualitative tests

Table 9 presents the results of the phytochemical tests. These tests reveal that the hydroethanolic extract (50/50, v/v) of S. longipedunculata leaves contains flavonoids, tannins, saponosides, alkaloids and carbohydrates.

Table 9: Results of chemical group identification tests

Groupes chimiques	Réactifs	Extrait de *S. longipedunculata*
Flavonoïdes	Chlorure ferrique 1%	+
	NaOH 1/10	+
Tannins	Chlorure ferrique 1%	+
Polyphénols	Chlorure ferrique 1%	+
Saponosides	Test de mousse	+
Alcaloïdes	Bouchardart (iode bisaublimé + iodure de potassium + eau)	+
	Dragendorf (Nitrate basique de Bismuth + acide acétique + eau)	+
		+
	Mayer (iode + iodure de potassium + eau)	
Glucides	Réactif de Molisch + H_2SO_4	+

2. Determination of flavonoids, total polyphenols and tannins

The total quantity of flavonoids or total phenols or tannins present in the extract of the leaves of S. longipedunculata expressed in milligram equivalent of rutin for flavonoids or gallic acid for phenolic compounds and tannins per gram of extract are recorded in **Figure 10**. Flavonoid content was determined using the equation $y = 0.0052x + 0.023$; $R^2 = 0.9981$ and polyphenol content using the equation $y = 0.0245x + 0.041$; $R^2 = 0.9983$.

Figure 10: Phytochemical content of the extract

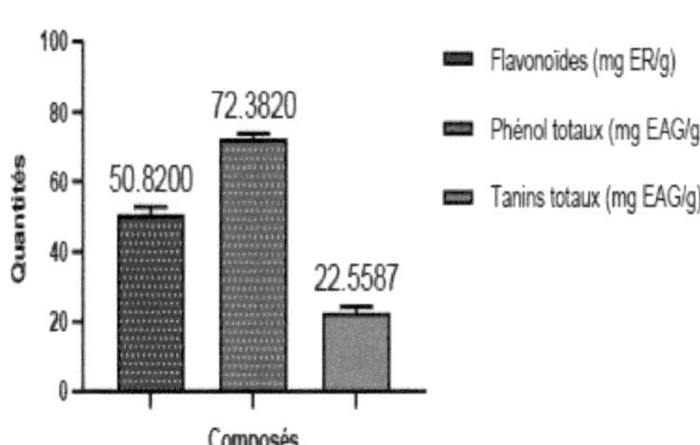

III. In vitro anti-inflammatory test

3.1. Egg albumin denaturation inhibition test

The CIs$_{50}$ for extract and diclofenac in the albumin denaturation inhibition test are shown in **Table 10**.

Table 10: Anti-inflammatory effect denaturation of egg albumin.	from	Securidaca longipedunculata on the
Substances		IC50 (μg/mL)
S.longipedunculata extract		99.87 ± 0.26
Diclofenac		49.54 ± 0.04

3.2. Membrane stabilisation tests

The IC values$_{50}$ for the extract and the standard (Aspirin) are shown in the table below. Table 11.

Table 11: Anti-inflammatory effect of Securidaca longipedunculata on membrane stabilisation of red blood cells.

SubstancesIC50 (µg/mL)

	Hypotonia	Heat
S.longipedunculata extract	305.657 ±0.133	471.75 ± 0.096
Aspirin	246.117 ± 1.055	368.743 ± 0.632

IV. In vitro antioxidant tests

4.1. Total antioxidant capacity (TAC) and DPPH

The antioxidant capacity of the extract and ascorbic acid as determined by phosphomolybdenum reduction and the percentage DPPH scavenging effect of the extract and ascorbic acid are shown in the table below.

Table 12: Antioxidant activity of Securidaca longipedunculata using TAC and DPPH tests.

Substances	TAC (mg EAG/g)	DPPH IC50 (µg/mL)
S.longipedunculata extract	97.83 ± 1.29	76.22 ± 0.02
Ascorbic acid		38.5 ± 0.04

4.2. Inhibition of lipoperoxidation

Figure 11: Effect of S. longipedunculata extract on lipoperoxidation in bone marrow.

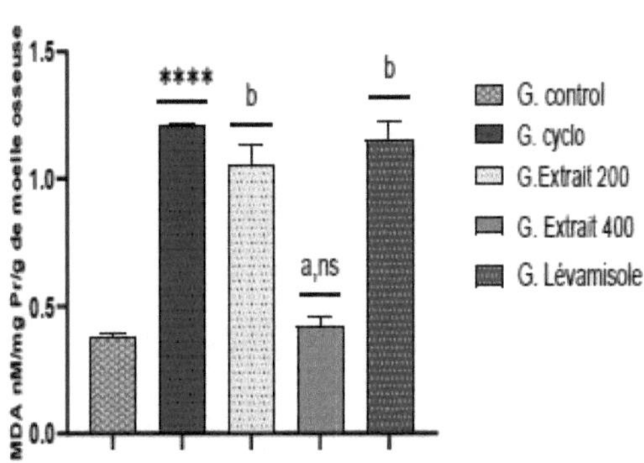

Results are expressed as means ± S.E.M.

(**** means very significant compared with G. Control p<0.0001; ns means no significant compared with G. Contro p<0.05;

a means significant compared with G. Cyclo p< 0.001; b means no significant compared with G. Cyclo P<0.05)

The MDA value in nM/mg Pr/g bone marrow increased significantly from 0.3923 ± 0.1110 in normal rats to 1.1979 ± 0.1101 in rats treated with cyclophosphamide. In rats treated with the 200mg/kg + cyclo and 400mg/kg + cyclo extracts the MDA doses were 1.1100 ± 0.550 and 0.4457 ± 0.02289 nM/mg Pr/g bone marrow respectively. There was a significant difference between the values for rats in the Cyclo group and those for rats treated with the 400mg/kg + cyclo extract. This value is 1.2072 ± 0.05364 nM/mg Pr/g bone marrow in rats. G. Levamisole rats, which was insignificant compared with that of G. Cyclo rats.

V. Immunomodulatory and anti-inflammatory activity of S. logipedunculata leaf extract in vivo Blood count (CBC)

Table 13: Titers of white blood cell types expressed as the number of cells per microlite of blood.

Cells	Control group	Cyclo Group	Group Extract 200mg/kg	Group Extract 400mg/kg	Levamisole group
Leukocytes	7280 ± 168	794 ± 140.7	876 ± 175.3	950 ± 169.9	1062 ± 274.2
Lymphocytes	3506 ± 100.5	476 ± 67.72	518 ± 130	580 ± 70.85	678 ± 150
Neutrophils	1738 ± 458	218 ± 55.80	244 ± 54.92	316 ± 82.79	160 ± 44.12
Basophile	366 ± 62.82	76 ± 28.74	90 ± 25.50	96 ± 32.19	88 ± 4
Monocytes	324 ± 13.02	10 ± 3.016	20 ± 10.49	60 ± 41.47b	52 ± 2

2. Determination of CRP

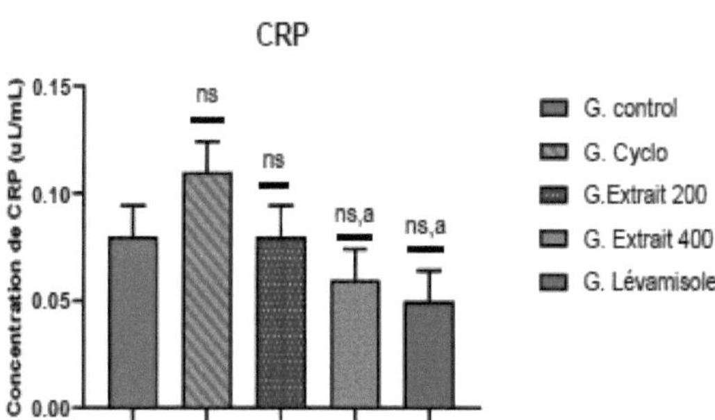

Figure 12: Influence of S. longipedunculata extract on CRP titre in rats. Results are expressed as means ± S.E.M.

(ns means no significant compared with G. Control; a means significant compared with G. Cyclo; P<0.05)

The CRP concentration increased from an average of 0.08 ± 0.02ul/mL in normal rats to 0.11 ± 0.01ul/mL in rats treated with cyclophosphamide. This represents an increase, although the difference was not significant between the two groups. The difference in mean CRP concentrations between rats treated with extract 200mg/kg + cyclo, extract 400mg/kg + cyclo and those treated with levamisole were 0.08 ± 0.01ul/mL; 0.06 ± 0.04ul/mL and 0.05 ± 0.02ul/mL respectively.

VI. Determination of lactate dehydrogenase LDH

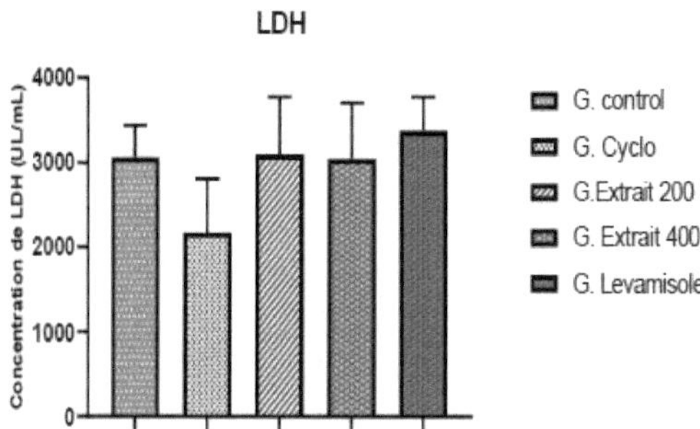

Figure 13: Influence of S. longipedunculata on LDH enzymatic activity in rats. Results are expressed as means ± S.E.M.

Concentrations of LDH enzyme activity in G. Control rats were was recorded as a mean of 3060 ± 169.9ul/ml. Rats treated with cyclophosphamide showed a mean concentration of 2167 ± 287.7ul/ml, which was not significantly different ($p < 0.05$) from that in the G. Control.Rats treated with the 200mg/kg + Cyclo and 400mg/kg + Cyclo extracts showed LDH concentrations of 3052 ± 613.3ul/ml and 3049 ± 293.9ul/ml respectively, which were not only significantly different from each other but also from the normal control group. Rats treated with levamisole hydrochloryde had a mean LDH dose equal to 3380 ± 613.3ul/ml, which was also non-significantly different compared with the other groups.

DISCUSSION

Extraction is the main step in the recovery and isolation of bioactive phytochemicals. It is influenced by the extraction process used, the particle size, the sample and the presence of interfering substances **(Stalikas, 2007).** The combined use of water and ethanol can facilitate the extraction of substances that are soluble in water and/or ethanol. In fact, the use of dry material for polyphenol extraction is recommended as flavonoids can undergo enzymatic degradation when plant material is fresh or undried **(Marston and Hostettmann, 2006)**. Microbial fermentation caused by humidity can also be the cause of this degradation. Drying in the dark prevents chemical transformations such as isomerisation and degradation caused by UV radiation from sunlight **(Jones and Kinghorn, 2005)**. The use of powder improves extraction because the contact surface between the sample and the solvent is greater, and penetration into cells not destroyed after grinding is easier. The yields calculated by **Dembélé et al (2022)**, **Dembele et al (2021)** and **Diakité (2016)** from a hydroethanolic extract of S. longipedunculata harvested in Kati (Mali) are 23.36%, 31.97% and 16.42% respectively. These yields are higher than the one we found before (15.05%). This variability in yields depends on several parameters such as: solvent, PH, temperature, time, extraction method, sample harvesting period, geographical origin of the plant, conditions and duration of storage of the harvest. The work carried out by **Odebiyi (1978)** showed the absence of flavonoids in the leaves of S. longipedunculata. Our study, on the other hand, revealed the presence of flavonoids in the leaves of S. longipedunculata. This could be due to the plant's geographical origin. Our study confirmed the immunosuppressive effect of cyclophosphamide administered on days 11^e , 12^e and 13^e to rats in the Cyclo group: leukopenia (p<0.001), lymphopenia (p<0.001), neutropenia (p<0.0001), hypobasophilia (p<0.001) and monocytopenia (p<0.05), as demonstrated in previous studies **(Bach, 1985; Guo et al, 2016)**. In addition, the 200mg/kg and 400mg/kg doses of S. longipedunculata extract administered to the G. Extract 200 and G. Extract 400 generally did not significantly boost the levels of these immune cells. If our analyses show in almost all cases a non-significant difference between the results of the groups of rats treated with S. longipedunculata extract (G. Extract 200 and G. Extract 400) and those treated with levamisole, which is known as an immunostimulant and used or cited by several authors in their studies as a reference immunostimulant **(Libeau and Pinder, 1981; Guo et al., 2016; Tibitondwa et al., 2018)**, then S. longipedunculata extract (G. Extract 200 and G. Extract 400) is the most effective immunostimulant. longipedunculata would have an immunostimulant effect similar to that of levamisole. It would be preferable to continue administering the extract alone to the rats for a further week or two after cyclophosphamide gavage, in order to clearly detect whether or not there was a clear difference between the values of the parameters measured in different treated batches. Indeed, cyclophosphamide has not only induced immunosuppression but also inflammation as a side effect **(Sevko et al., 2013; ANSM, 2017)**; and that in our study the extract of S. longipedunculata would have played an anti-inflammatory activity given that the types of leukocytes whose titer we measured participate actively in inflammatory reactions. It is in this line of activity that the results of the hen egg albumin denaturation inhibition and membrane stabilisation tests; supported by those of C-Reactive Protein (CRP), which is a very good marker of the acute phase of inflammation **(Engler, 1995 ; Wilwert, 2008)**, obtained from analyses carried out on blood sera from the same animals as those used for blood cell count (CBC) analyses, provide further evidence of the anti-inflammatory activity of S. longipedunculata coupled with its immunomodulatory activity. In fact, inflammation is an integral part of immunity and our study is further proof of this. In fact, the CRP results show that the S. longipedunculata extract reduced the inflammation caused by cyclophosphamide; this was reflected by the reduction in CRP concentration from 0.11 ± 0.01uL/mL (G. Cyclo) to 0.08 ± 0.01uL/mL (G. Extract 200) and 0.06 ± 0.04uL/mL (G. Extract 400). These results show that S. longipedunculata stimulated the inflammation caused by cyclophosphamide. longipedunculata would have stimulated the bone marrow to produce leukocytes and would have protected the cells against the chemical and enzymatic modifications induced by the immunosuppressive agent; and at the same time limit the inflammatory response by curbing the production of autoantigens, which would also relieve the organ damage caused by the inflammatory processes **(Woolbright, 2020).** Also during inflammation, lysosomal enzymes such as bactericidal enzymes and proteases are released and several typical alterations can occur **(Saleem et al., 2020).** Lysosomal membrane stabilisation is important for limiting the inflammatory response by preventing the release of lysosomal constituents from activated neutrophils, which cause further tissue inflammation when released extracellularly. The membranes of erythrocytes and lysosomes are similar so the membrane stabilisation of red blood cells could be extrapolated to the membrane stabilisation of lysosomes **(Agarwal et al, 2019, Anosike et al, 2012).** The anti-inflammatory activity of levamisole is also revealed by our study as the difference between the CRP values of the G. Cyclo group and that of G. Levamisole is significant ($p<0.05$). Extract at 400mg/kg and levamisole at 30mg/kg would have been sufficient in the our study to significantly prevent hepatocytes from releasing CRP, which has the biological functions of activating the complement system, stimulating phagocytosis and opsonisation. Our extract also has antioxidant activity. We observed a highly significant ($p < 0.0001$) increase in MDA in rats receiving cyclophosphamide and not treated (0.3923 ± 0.1110 nM/mg Pr/g bone marrow) compared with the normal control group (1.1979 ± 0.1101 nM/mg Pr/g bone marrow). The extract administered at a dose of 200mg/kg did not significantly reduce the MDA value compared with the group of rats treated with cyclophosphamide alone. Furthermore, no significant variation in MDA was observed in rats receiving cyclophosphamide and pre-treated with S. longipedunculata extract at a dose of 400mg/kg (its value of 0.4457 ± 0.02289 nM/mg Pr/g bone marrow was not significantly different from that obtained with the normal control, $p<0.05$). These results, supported by those of the CAT and DPPH tests, probably explain the protection of the animals by S. longipedunculata extract against oxidative stress. It could be that cyclophosphamide, which is an alkylating agent, produced free radicals that interacted directly with the DNA of bone marrow cells in G0 phase by forming covalent bonds with the nucleophilic substrate, resulting in cell destruction by inhibiting DNA transcription and replication. In short, cyclophosphamide would have caused bone marrow aplasia. This could prevent the rapid proliferation of haematopoietic stem cells and, consequently, the slow immunostimulant effect of S. longipedunculata extract. The MDA value obtained in rats receiving cyclophosphamide and pretreated with levamisole (1.2072 ± 0.05364 nM/mg Pr/g bone marrow) was not significant compared with the MDA value in rats treated with cyclophosphamide alone. This proves that levamisole probably does not inhibit lipid peroxidation and that its immunostimulant mechanism is distinct from that of our extract. The antioxidant effect is due to natural compounds, in particular the polyphenols and flavonoids present in our extract. According to **Halliwell (1994)**, polyphenols exert their antioxidant power through various mechanisms, the main ones being: direct scavenging of ROS, chelation of metal ions that initiate ROS production and direct inhibition of enzymes involved in oxidative stress or their transcription. On the other hand, the lactate dehydrogenase enzyme assay, which averaged 3060±169.9IU/ml in normal rats and 2167±287.7IU/ml in rats treated with cyclophosphamide proves that cyclophosphamide reduced the energy activity of the cells. Meanwhile, the LDH results obtained in the groups treated with 200mg/kg and 400mg/kg of extract, which were 3052±613.3IU/ml and 3049±293.9IU/ml respectively, were not significant compared with the normal group. This shows that the S. longipedunculata extract restored the lactate/pyruvate (L/P) ratio, thereby ensuring energy balance in the cells. Our extract is thought to have a cytoprotective effect. Not only did S. longipedunculata extract promote the production of leukocytes, but these cells will also have the energy they need to vigorously carry out their role in defending the body.

CONCLUSION AND OUTLOOK

Securidaca longipedunculata is a plant widely used in traditional medicine and pharmacology. The present study involved evaluating the immunomodulatory and anti-inflammatory activity of the hydroethanol extract (50/50, v/v) of Securidaca longipedunculata leaves. The results of the assay of the parameters studied are evidence that the hydroalcoholic extract has potential immunostimulant, anti-inflammatory, antioxidant and cytoprotective activities, and should encourage the scientific world to pursue immunomodulatory research on S. longipedunculata in order to save mankind, which is constantly faced with diseases linked to immunological disorders. We therefore envisage the following perspectives:

- Continue to treat the animals with the extract until 21^e or 28^e day.
- Blood samples were taken before and just after the animals were gavaged with cyclophosphamide (10^e and 14^e days) and at 21^e or 28^e day.
- Use doses higher than 400mg/kg
- Use extracts obtained by maceration of different mixtures: Volume-water/Volume-alcohol (ethanol, methanol, buthanol).
- Perform other immunomodulation tests such as: determination of the phagocytic index, serum haemolysis rate and delayed-type hypersensitivity (DTH).
- Use other immunosuppressants such as corticosteroids.

BIBLIOGRAPHICAL REFERENCES

Adebiyi R. A., Elsa A. T., Agaie B. M, Etuk E.U., 2006. Antinoceptive and antidepressant like effects of Securidaca longependunculata root extract in mice. Journal of Ethnopharmacology 107: 234 - 239

Agarwal Happy, Amatullah Nakara, Venkat Kumar Shanmugam, 2019. Anti-inflammatory mechanism of various metal and metal oxide nanoparticles synthesized using plants extracts: A review. Biomed Pharmacother. doi: 10.1016/j.biopha.2018.11.116.

Alexandre D. Y, 2002. Initiation à l'agroforesterie en zone sahélienne. Ed. Karthala, p 154.

Almagboul. A.Z, Farouk. A, Bashir. A.K, Karim. A, Salah. M, 1985. Antibacterial activity of Sudanese plants used in folkloric Medicine III. Phytotherapy 56, 195-200.

Amjad Ali Khan, Khaled S. Allemailem, Fahad Abdulrahman Alhumaydhi, Sivakumar J T Gowder, Arshad Husain Rahmani, 2019. The Biochemical and Clinical Perspectives of Lactate Dehydrogenase: An Enzyme of Active Metabolism. Bentham Science Publishers/Endocrine, Metabolic & Immune Disorders - Drug Targets, 2020, Vol. 20, No. 00. DOI: 10.2174/1871530320666191230141110

Anosike C.A, Obidoa O, Ezeanyika L.U., 2012. Membrane stabilization as a mechanism of the anti-inflammatory activity of methanol extract of garden egg (Solanum aethiopicum). Daru Journal of Pharmaceutical Sciences, 20 : 76

ANSM (Agence Nationale de Sécurité du Médicament), 2017. Summary of Product Characteristics. Available at http://agence-prd.ansm.santé.fr. Accessed on 24 December 2022.

Aouissa Itian, W.R. (2002). Etudes des activités biologiques et de la toxicité aigüe de l'extrait aqueux des feuilles de Mangifera indica (Anacardiaceae) ;

thèse doctorale université de Bamako, P : 48.

Athamena, S., Chalghem1, I., Kassah-Laouar, A., Laroui, S., Khebri, S., (2010). Antioxidant and antimicrobial activity of extracts of Cuminum cyminum l. Lebanese Science Journal, 11(1) :69-81.

Auwal SM, Atiku Mk, Alhassan Muhammad Wudil, Mohamed Sani Sule, 2012. Phytochemical composition and acute toxicity evaluation of Securidaca longipedunculata (Linn) aqueous root bark extract. Bayero Journal of Pure and Applied Sciences Vol. 5 n ° 2 : 67-72. DOI : 10.4314/bajopas. v5i2.12.

Bach J.F., 1985. Immune deficiency induced by immunosuppressants. Médecine et Maladies Infectieuses -- 1985 -- 5 - 251 & 254.

Baggnian Issoufou, Abdou Laouali, Yamego Jérôme, Moussa Ibrahima, Adam Toudou. 2018. Ethnobotanical study of medicinal plants sold in markets in west-central Niger. Journal of Applied Biosciences 132: 13392- 13403 ISSN 1997-5902. J. Appl. Biosci. https://dx.doi.org/10.4314/jab.v132i1.1 Published online at www.m.elewa.org on 31st December 2018.

Bah. S, Jäger. AK, Adsersen. A, Diallo. D, Paulsen. BS, 2007. Antiplasmodial and GABAbenzodiazepin receptor buding actvities of five plants used in traditional medicine in Mali. West Africa, Journal of ethnopharmacology, 110(13): 451-757.

Beaulieu Josée, 2008. Immunomodulatory and anti-inflammatory effect of a malleable protein matrix (MPM) derived from the fermentation of whey by Lactobacillus Kefiranofaciens subsp. R2C2. INRS-Institut Armand Frappier, Thesis submitted for the degree of philosophiae doctor (Ph. D.) in virology and immunology, 2008.

Beuscher N, Bodinet C, Neumann-Haefelim D, Marstom A, Hostettmann. K, 1994. Antiviral activity of African medicinal plants. Jounal ethnopharmacology, 42, 101-109.

Birben, E., Sahiner, U.M., Sackesen,C., Serpil,E., Kalayci,o., 2012. Oxidative

Stress and Antioxidant Defense. WAO Journal, 5, 9-19.

Birben, E., Sahiner, U.M., Sackesen, C., Serpil, E., Kalayci, O., 2012. Oxidative Stress and Antioxidant Defense. WAO Journal, 5, 9-19.

Buxton T., V.Y.Eziah, E.O. Owusu, 2014. Bio-activities of Powders of four plants against Prostephanus truncatus Horn. (Coleoptera: Bostrichidae) and Tribolium Castaneum Herbst (Coleoptera: Tenebrionidae). WestAfrican Journal ofAppliedEcology, vol. 22 (1), 2014.

Causse, C., (1994). Les secrètes de santé des antioxydants: les antioxydants faits maison. 7éd. Monaco, 16-18.

Cemerski S, Shaw A, 2006. Immune synapses in T-cell activation. Curr Opin Immunol : 18(3):298-304. doi: 10.1016/j.coi.2006.03.011. Epub 2006 Apr 17. PMID : 16603343.

Chatenoud, L, 2002. Cells of immunity. In: Immunology, from biology to the clinic. J. F. Bach and L. Chatenoud. Paris, France: Flammarion Médicine-Sciences. 369 p.

CNPM (Collège National de Pharmacologie Médicale), 2018. Corticosteroids: Essential points. Available at https://pharmacomedicale.org

Cohen, R., Romain, O., Levy, C., Perreaux, F., Decobert, M., Hau, I., Lécuyer,.A, Lesprit,E., Maman, L., Roullaud, S., 1981. Impact of C-reactive protein (CRP). Arch Ped, P: 13-38.

CoPath (French College of Pathologists), 2011. The inflammatory reaction.

Costa C., Bortazzo A., Allegri G., Curcuroto D., Traloli P., 1992. Indole alkaloids from the roots on an African plant, Securidaca longipedunculata. Isolation by column chromatography and preliminary structural characterization by mass spectrometry. Journal heterocycle. Chemestry. P : 1641-1647.

Davoust-Nataf Nathalie, 2021. Innate immunity: Natural barriers and inflammatory response. CIRI (Centre International de Recherche en

Infectiologie), Lyon. Available at www.acces.ens-lyon.fr. Accessed on 24 December 2021.

Debne, 1999. Africa reprod health 1999; 3(2): 40-50

Declaude, C., 1971. Comparative study of saponins extracted from two African Polygalaceae: Securidaca longipedunculata Fres and Polygala aciculans. Bulletin soc. Royal des sciences. Liège (397-405).

Dembélé D.L., Haidara M., Denou A & Sanogo R., 2021. Etude phytochimique des écorce de Racines et des Feuilles de Securidaca Longipedunculata (Fresen), Polygalaceae Au Mali. European Scientific Journal, ESJ, 17(29), 145. https://doi.org/10.19044/esj.2021.v17n29p145

Dembélé Daouda Lassine, Denou Adama, Haidara Mahamane, Sanogo Rokia, 2022. Formulation of analgesic and anti-inflammatory ointment based on Securidaca longipedunculata Fresen (Polygalaceae). Journal of the Cameroon academy of sciences Vol. 17 No. 3

Diakité Bréhima, 2008. The susceptibility of Anopheles gambiae larvae to medicinal plant extracts from Mali. UNIVERSITY OF BAMAKO. Thesis presented and publicly defended on 28/03/2008 before the Faculty of Medicine, Pharmacy and Odonto Stomatology. To obtain the degree of Doctor of Medicine (state diploma)

Dosseh K., Kpatcha T., Adjrah Y., Idoh K., Agbonon A. & Gbeassor M., 2014. Antiinflammatory effect of Byrsocarpus schum. And thonn. (connaraceae) root. World journal of pharmaceutical Reseach, 3(3), 14.

Eldeen I.M., Staden J.Van, 2008. Cyclooxygenase inhibition and antimycobacterial effects of extracts from Sudanese medicinal plants. Research Center for Plant Growth and Development, School of Biological and Conservation Sciences, University of Kwazulu-Natal Pietermaritzburg, Private Bag x01, Scoottsville 3209, South Africa. Edited by JN Eloff.

Ellyard, J.I., Simson, L., and Parish, C.R., 2007. Th2-mediated anti-tumour immunity: friend or foe? Tissue Antigens 70, 1-11

Elufioye T., Alafe A., Faborode O. Moody J., 2014. Anti-Inflammatory and Analgesic Activities of Securidaca longipedunculata Fers (Polygalaceae) Leaf and Stem Bark Methanolic Extract. Afr. J. Biomed. Res. Vol.17 : 187-191.

Engler R., 1995. Protein of the inflammatory reaction. Revue françaie des labratoires. Volume 1995, Issue 276. Pages 93-99. https://doi.org/10.1016/S0338-9898(95)80365-3

Favier, A., 2003. Le stress oxydant, interet conceptuel et experimental dans la compréhension des mecanismes des maladies et potentiel therapeutique. L'actualité Chimique, 11, 108-115.

Ferran Aude, 2013. Glucocorticoids and corticosteroid therapy in domestic animals. Ecole Nationale de Vétérinaire (ENV), Toulouse. Edited by Dorothée Larrivée. Available at https://slidesplayer.fr

Fletcher MA, Klimas A, Morgan R, Gjereet G., 1992. Lymphocyte Proliferation. In Manual of Clinical Laboratory Immunology. American Association for Microbiology. New York. pp. 213-219

Garba Abdoul Razak Issa, Adakal Hassane, Abasse Tougiani, Koudouvo Koffi, Karim Saley, Akourki Adamou, Gbeassor Messanvi, Mahamane Saadou, 2019. Ethnobotanical studies of plants used in the treatment of digestive parasitosis of small ruminants (sheep) in Southwest Niger. http://www.ifgdg.org Int. J. Biol. Chem. Sci. 13(3): 1534-1546.

Gardès-Albert, M., Abedinzadeh, Z., Jore, D., 2003. Reactive oxygen species: how can oxygen become toxic? Le journal de la société chimique en France (L'actualité chmique), (270), 91-96.

Gloaguen Daniel, 2007. C-reactive protein (CRP), a highly sensitive inflammatory index. Masine Belle-santé N°095. Available at www.belle-sante.com

Gordon Chalmers, 2017. What are immunostimulants. Available at https://www.aviators-loft.com. Accessed 22 January 2022.

Gruffat Xavier, 2021. Inflammation. From the October 2020 issue of the Newsletter of Havard Medical School on chronic inflammation, updated on 14 September 2021. Available at www.ceapharma.ch

Guo Ze, Hong-Yan Xu, Lu Xu, Sha-Sha Wang, Xue-Mei Zhang, 2016. In vivo and in vitro imunomodulatry and antiinflammatory effects of total flavonoides as Astragalus. Afr J Tradit Complement Altern Med. (2016) 13(4):60-73 doi:10.21010/ajtcam. v13i4.10 60

Halliwell, B., Cross-, C. E., 1994. Oxygen-derived species: their relation to human disease and environmental stress. Environmental health perspectives, 102(Suppl 10), 5.

Javed, F., Jabeen, Q., Aslam, N. and Awan, A. M., 2020. "Pharmacological evaluation of analgesic, anti-inflammatory ant antipyretic activities of ethanolique extract of Indigofera argenta Burm. F." Ehnopharmacol. 259 : 29-66.

Jayasekara, TK, Stevenson, PC, Hall, DR, 2005. Effect of volatile constituents of Securidaca Longipedunculata on insect pests of stored grain. J Chem Ecol 31, 303-313. https://doi.org/10.1007/s10886-005-1342-0

Jiofack T., Fokunang C., Guedje N., Kemeuze V., Fonnossie E, Nkongmeneck B. A., Mapongmetsem P. M. and Tsabang N., 2010. Ethnobotanical uses of medicinal plants of two ethnoecological regions of Cameroon. International Journal of Medicine and Medical Sciences 2(3): 60-79.

Jones Paul Guillaume, Kingborn Douglas Un, 2012. Extraction of plant Secondary Metabolites. Methods in molecular biology (Clifton, N.J.) 624:341-66. DOI:10.1007/978-1-61779-624-1_13. Source PubMed.

Joseph, Moshi, Sympombe, Nkunya, 2006. African Journal of traditional medicine, vol3, n°3, Pp: 80:86. Bioline, 2006.

Junaid S. A, Abubakar A.,Ofodile, A. C., Olabode A. O.,Echeonwu, G. O. N., Okwori
A. E. J., Adetunji J. A., 2008. Evaluation of Securidaca longipenduculata leaf and root extracts for antimicrobial activities. African Journal of Microbiology Research 2: 322- 325.

Juneau Martin, 2017. Non-steroidal anti-inflammatory drugs and cardiovascular risk. Montreal Heart Institute, Faculty of Medicine, Université de Montréal. Available at https://observatoireprevention.org

Kalam S., Gul M.Z., Singh R., Ankati S., 2015. Free radicals: Implications in etiology of chronic diseases and their amelioration through nutraceuticals. Pharmacologia. 6(1), 11-20.

Kara A. W., 2018. Effect of extracts from the medicinal plant Ruta montana. Biology
Thèse de doctorat d'état, Université de Constantine, Algérie, 126p

Kayode AAA, MA Sonibaré, Jo Moody, 2015. Antiulcer activities of Securidaca longipedunculata Fres. (Polygalaceae) and Luffa cylindrica Linn. (Cucurbits) in Wistar rats. Vol. 19. DOI : 10.4314/njnpm. v19i0.9

Kerharo. J, Adam, 1974. La pharmacopée Sénégalaise traditionnelle: Plantes médicinales et toxiques. Edition Vigot et Frères, Paris, 1011 pages.

Koechlin-Ramonatxo, C., 2006. Oxygen, oxidative stress and antioxidant supplementation or a different aspect of nutrition in respiratory disease. Nutrition Clinique & Métabolisme, 20, 165 - 177.

Kola P., Metowogo K., Manjula S. N., Katawa G., Elkhenany H., Mruthunjaya K. M., Eklu-Gadegbeku K., Aklikokou K. A., 2022. Ethnopharmacological evaluation of antioxidant, anti-angiogenic, and anti-inflammatory activity of some traditional medicinal plants used for treatment of cancer in Togo/Africa. Journal of Ethnopharmacology 283 (2022) 114673. https://doi.org/10.1016/j.jep.2021.114673

Kone Kéassemon Hervé Cédessia, Coulibaly Kiyinlma; Konan Kouakou Severin, 2019. Identification of some plants used in ethnoveterinary medicine in Sinématiali (Northern Ivory Coast). Journal of Applied Biosciences 135: 13766 - 13774 ISSN 1997-5902. https://dx.doi.org/10.4314/jab.v135i1.3

Kpemissi, M., Eklu-Gadegbeku, K., Veerapur, V. P., Potârniche, A-V., Adi, K., Vijayakumar S., Banakar, S. M., Thimmaiah, N. V., Metowogo, K., and Aklikokou, K., 2019b. Antioxidant and nephroprotection activities of Combretum micranthum: A phytochemical, in vitro and ex-vivo studies. Heliyon 5(3): e01365.

Kpoyizoun Pascaline Kindji, Metowogo Kossi, Kantati Yendoube, Missebukpo Afiwa, Dare Thin, Lawson-Evi Povi, Eklu-Gadegbeku Kwashie, Aklikokou Kodjo, 2020. Antiinflammatory and antioxidant evaluation of Maytenus senegalensis hydroalcoholic roots extract fractions in allergic asthma. JPHYTO 2020; 9(4): 252-257

Laurent PE., 1988. Induction and regulation of the systemic inflammatory reaction. Ann Biol Clin (Paris). 1988 ;46(5):329-35. French. PMID : 3138927.

Lawin Iboukoun Fidèle, Laleye Obafemi Arnauld Fernand and Agbani Onodjè Pierre, 2016. Vulnerability and endogenous conservation strategies for plants used in the treatment of diabetes in the communes of Glazoué and Savè in Centre-Bénin. Available online at http://www.ifg-dg.org Int. J. Biol. Chem. Sci. 10(3): 1069-1085.

Lenz. W., 1913. Un tersuchungen der wurzelrin de von Securidaca longipedunculata. Arbeiten aus dem Pharm. Inst.D. Univ. Berlin, 10, 177-180.

Li, H., and Rostami, A., 2010. IL-9: basic biology, signaling pathways in CD4+ T cells and implications for autoimmunity. J Neuroimmune Pharmacol 5, 198-

209

Libeau G., Pinder M., 1981. Detrimental effect of levamisole on experimental trypanosomosis in mice. Rev. Elev. Méd. vét. Pays trop, 1981, 34 (4): 399-404.

Ma, Q.-Y., Huang, D.-Y., Zhang, H.-J., Chen, J., Miller, W., and Chen, X.-F., 2016. Function of follicular helper T cell is impaired and correlates with survival time in non-small cell lung cancer. Int. Immunopharmacol. 41, 1-7

Mahamood. N, Moore. P.S, De Tommasi. N, De Simone. F, Colman. S, Hay. A.J, Pizza. C, 1993. Inhibition of H.I.V infection by caffeoyquinic acid derivatives isolate from securidaca longipedunculata roots. Antiviral Chem Chemother. 235-240.

Malagas D., 1992. Arbres et arbustes guérisseurs des savanes Maliennes. ACCT - Karthala, p. 232.

Malaise F., 1992. La gestion des produits sauvages comestibles, Défis-sud, 7: 18-19.

Manciaux M.A., 1993. Thérapeutiques médicamenteuses en gériatrie. Anti-inflammatoires non stéroïdiens et antalgiques. Ed Masson 1993: 115-118.

Marston Andrew, Hostettmann Kurt, 2006. Separation and quantification of flavonoids/ Flavonoids: chemistry, biochemistry and applications, pp.1-36. Ref.113. CRC Press LLC. Available at www.caddirect.org

Mathias. M.E, 1982. Some medicinal plants of hehe (Southern Highland Province, Tanzania) Taxon 31, 488-494.

Mbaihougadobe Séverin, Ngakebni-limbili Adolphe Christian, Gouollaly Tsiba, Ngaissona Paul, Koane Jean Noel, Nkounkou Loumpangou Célestine, Mahmout Yaya and Ouamba Jean Maurille, 2017. Inventory and phytochemical tests on some plants from Chad used in the treatment of gout. J. Biol. Chem. Sci. 11(6): 2693-2703. https://dx.doi.org/10.4314/ijbcs.v11i6.11

Meunier Lucy, Dominique Larrey, 2018. Update on the hepatotoxicity of non-steroidal anti-inflammatory drugs. Hôpital Saint Eloi, Service d'hépatogastroentérologie et transplantation, 80 avenue Fliche, 34295 Montpellier Cedex 5, France 2 INSERM.1183. P.239.

Meyer JJ, Rakuambo NC, Hussein AA. 2008. Novel xanthones from Securidaca longipedunculata with activity against erectile dysfunction. J Ethnopharmacol. 2008 Oct 28;119(3):599-603. doi: 10.1016/j.jep.2008.06.018. Epub 2008 Jun 27. PMID:18638534.

.Mirandole, 2020. Difference between innate and adaptive immunity. Available at www.jeretiens.net

Morelon Emmanuel, 2001. Les rapamycines, nouveaux immunosuppresseurs : des mécanismes d'action aux applications cliniques. Therapeutic Medicine. 2001;7(2):152-6.

Mury Pauline, 2018. Mechanism and impact of physical activity and sedentarisation on biological risk factors for carotid atherosclerotic plaque instability. PhD thesis, May 2018. LIBM (Laboratoire Interuniversitaire de Biologie de la Motricité); Physiology, University of Lyon. Available at https://archives-ouvertes.fr/tel-01878197. Submitted on Thursday 20 September 2018(17 :51 :06), modified on Friday 06 November 2020-03 :31 :44, Archived to long expired on Friday 21 December 2018-16 :08 :12. Accessed on 24 December 2021.

Namadina, M. M., Shawai, R. S., Musa, F. M., Sunusi, U., Aminu, M. A., Nuhu, Y. and Umar, A. M., 2020. Phytochemical and Antimicrobial Activity of Securidaca longipedunculata Root against Urinary Tract Infection Pathogens. CSJ 11(2): 2276 - 2707.

Ndou Avhuverengwi Phillemon, 2006. Monograph of Securidaca longipedunculata Fresen. Watter sisuli national botanic garden, august 2006.

Nuhrich Alain, 2015. Non-steroidal anti-inflammatory drugs (NSAIDs). UFR

(Unité de Formation de Recherche) des Sciences Pharmacologiques, University of Bordeaux. Available at http://unt-ori2.crihan.fr.

Odebiyi. O.O, 1978. Preliminary phytochemical and antimicrobial examination of leaves of Securidaca longipedunculata Fresen. Niger. Journal Pharmaceutic, 9, 29-30.

Ojewole J., Ilesanmi O., Gbola O., 2000. Pharmacology of African medicinal plants: Neuromuscular and cardiovascular properties of Securidaca longipedunculata. Nig. J.Nat Prod. Vol.4 2000 :30-36.

Okoli CO, 2006. Anti-inflammatory activity of Securidaca longipedunculata fres (polygalaceae) root bark extracts. African Journal of Traditional, Complementary and Alternative Medicines Vol. 3(1) 2006: 54-63 Published 2005-12-15
Publish Vol. 3 No. 1.

WHO AFR/RC (World Health Organization, Regional Committee for Africa), 2000. Promoting the role of traditional medicine in health systems: strategy for the African region. Report of the Regional Director of the fiftieth session 28 August- 02 September 2000. Ouagadoudou, Burkina Faso.

WAHO (West African Health Organization), 2013. West African Pharmacopoeia. Designed, printed and bound by KS PRINTCRAFT GH. LTD.

Parameswari P., Devika R, Vijayaraghavan P. In vitro anti-inflammatory and antimicrobial potential of leaf extract from Artemisia nilagirica (Clarke) Pamp. Saudi Journal of Biological Sciences 26 (2019) 460-463. https://doi.org/10.1016/j.sjbs.2018.09.005

Petrovska Biljana Bauer, 2012. Historical review of medicinal plants' usage. National Institutes of Health.

Picard B and Bauchart D., 2010. Ruminant muscle and meat. Editions Quae. PP : 275.

Poprac P., Jomova K., Simunkova M., Kollar V., Rhodes C.J., Valko M. (2017). Targeting free radicals in oxidative stress-related human diseases. Trends in pharmacological sciences. 38(7), 592-607.

R Engler. Proteins of the inflammatory response, 1993. Veterinary Research vol 24 (4), pp.337-343. ffhal-00902134

Rasamindrakotroka Andry, 2013. Anti-inflammatory molecules. Faculty of Medicine, University of Antananarivo Madagascar. Available on www.andryrasamindrakotroka.e-monsite.com

Revillard, J.-P., 2001. Immunologie. Brussels, Belgium: De Boeck Université.595 p.

Rousselet, M.C., Vignaud, J. M., Hofman, P., Chatelet, F.P., 2005. Inflammation and inflammatory pathology. Edition AFECAP. P : 4-7.

Sadok, G., 2008. Phytotherapy. Magister thesis; hydro-thermo- thalassotherapy, Ecole Supérieure des Sciences et Techniques de la Santé de SOUSSE. P: 3.

Sagrawat H, Khan Y., 2007. Immunomodulatory Plants. A Phytopharmacological Review. Pharmacognosy Reviews 1: 248-260.

Saleem, A., Saleem, M., Akhtar, M.F., 2020. Antioxidant, anti-inflammatory and antiarthritic potential of Moringa oleifera Lam: an ethnomedicinal plant of Moringaceae family. South Afr. J. Bot. 128, 246-256. https://doi.org/10.1016/j.sajb.2019.11.023

Salhi S., Fadli M., Zidane L. & Douira A., 2010. Floristic and ethnobotanical studies of medicinal plants in the city of Kénitra (Morocco). Lazoroa 31: 133-146

Sevko A, Sade-Feldman M, Kanterman J, Michels T, Falk CS, Umansky L, Ramacher M, Kato M, Schadendorf D, Baniyash M, Umansky V., 2013. Cyclophosphamide promotes chronic inflammation-dependent immunosuppression and prevents antitumor response in melanoma. J Invest

Dermatol. 2013 Jun;133(6):1610-9. doi: 10.1038/jid.2012.444. Epub 2012 Dec 6. PMID: 23223128.

Sigal LH., 2005. Basic science for the clinician 30: The immunologic synapse. J Clin Rheumatol: 11(4):234-9. doi: 10.1097/01.rhu.0000173619.23349.09. PMID: 16357766.

Stalikas Constantine D, 2007. Extraction, separation, and detection methods for phenolic acids and flavonoids. J. Sep. Sci: 30, 3268 - 3295. DOI 10.1002/jssc.200700261.

Sylla Youssouf, Kone Witabouna Mamidou, Dieudonné Kigbafori Sillue, Kigninma Ouattara, 2018. Ethnobotanical study of plants used against malaria by traditherapists and herbalists in the district of Abidjan (Côte d'Ivoire). Available online at http://www.ifgdg.org

Tauheed Abdullah Mohammad, Mohammed Musa Suleiman, Mohamed Mamman Idris and Ala Lawal, 2017. Ex vivo trypanostatic effect of Securidaca longipedunculata (Fres. Holl) stem bark extracts against Trypanosoma brucei brucei. SOKOTO Journal of veterinarysciences 15(3): 78-84. DOI: 10.5897/AJB2015.14938.

Thomas boulanger, 2017. Pharmacology of anti-inflammatory drugs. IFSI, 06 December 2017.

Tibitondwa Josephine, Kokas Ikwap, Andrew Tamale, Gabriel Tumwine, John Kateregga, Samuel P. Wamala, Charles D. Kato, 2018. Immunomodulatory activity of the Chenopodium opulifolium total crude extract in wistar albino rats. Afr J Tradit Complement Altern Med, vol 15 (2) : 96-102 https://doi.org/10.21010/ajtcam.v15i2.12.

Tiksa Tahir, Dele Abdissa and Negera Abdissa, 2019. Chemical constituents of Securidaca longipedunculata root bark and evaluation of their antibacterial activities. Ethiopian Journal of Education and Science: Vol. 14 No. 2 / page 1-8.

Togashi, Y., Shitara, K., and Nishikawa, H., 2019. Regulatory T cells in cancer immunosuppression: implications for anticancer therapy. Nature Reviews Clinical Oncology 16, 356-371

Tolo. D., 2001. Etude des activités biologiques et de la toxicité des écorces de racines de Securidaca longipedunculata Fresen ; Thèse de Doctorat en pharmacie - Bamako, 110 pages.

Vane J.R., 1971. Inhibition of prostaglandin synthesis as a mechanim of action of aspirin-like drugs. Nature New Biol 1971; 231: 232-5.

Vidal, 2010. Guide to plants that heal. https://www.vidal.fr

Wannang Noel N, Alhassan M Wudil, Maxwell LP Dapar, Lawal A Bichi, 2006. Evaluation of anti-snake venom activity of the aqueous root extract of Securidaca longipedunculata in rats. Jounal of pharmacy & Bioressouces 2(2). DOI: 10.4314/jpb. v2i2.32067

Wilwert Ernest, Dourson Jean-Luc, Rausch Siggy, Weber Bernard, 2008. Biological markers of inflammation Short version Version 1.2 27.02.2008. 2 pages.

Woolbright, B. L., 2020. "Inflammation: cause or consequence of chronic cholestatic liver injury" Food Chem Toxicol 137: 111133.

Zerbato Mélina, 2010. The value of micromethod assay of C-reactive protein in paediatric practices. THESIS, presented and publicly defended on 28 January 2010 to obtain the Diplôme d'Etat de Docteur en Pharmacie. FACULTÉ DE PHARMACIE/ UNIVERSITÉ HENRI POINCARÉ - NANCY 1.

Zerbo P., J. Millogo-Rasolodimby, Nacoulma-Ouedraogo O. G., P. Van Damme P., 2007. Contribution à la connaissance des plantes médicinales utilisées dans les soins infantiles en pays San, au Burkina Faso. Int. J. Biol. Chem. Sci. 1(3): 262-274, 2007 ISSN 1991-8631. Available online at http://www.ajol.info

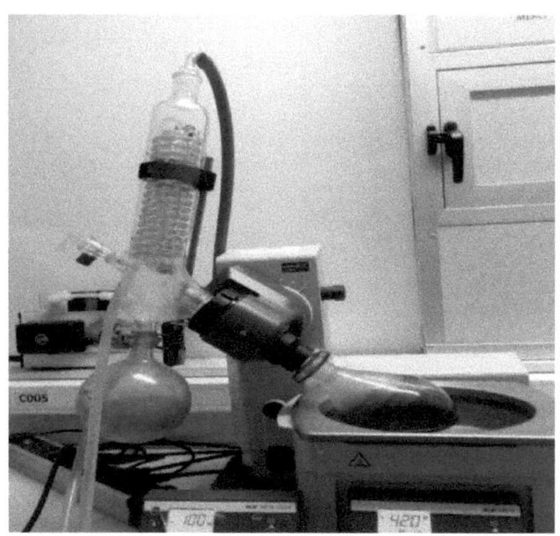

Photo 3: Rotavapeur (Source: Photograph, KPORVIE Atsu, 16 August 2022).

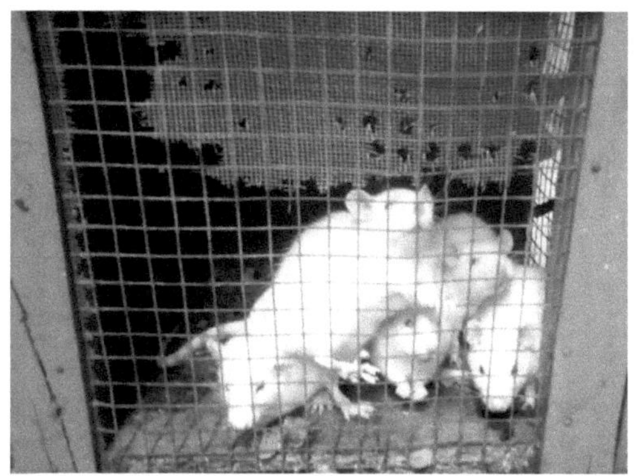

Photo 4: Sprague-dawley rats (Source: Photograph, KPORVIE Atsu, 02 December 2022).

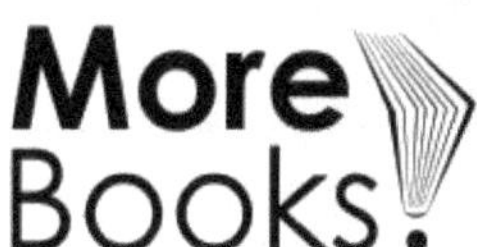

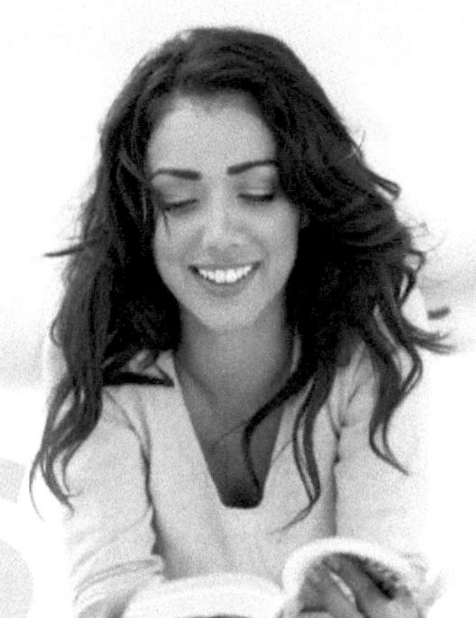

I want morebooks!

Buy your books fast and straightforward online - at one of world's fastest growing online book stores! Environmentally sound due to Print-on-Demand technologies.

Buy your books online at
www.morebooks.shop

Kaufen Sie Ihre Bücher schnell und unkompliziert online – auf einer der am schnellsten wachsenden Buchhandelsplattformen weltweit! Dank Print-On-Demand umwelt- und ressourcenschonend produzi ert.

Bücher schneller online kaufen
www.morebooks.shop

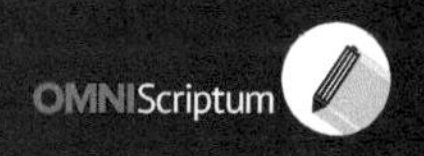

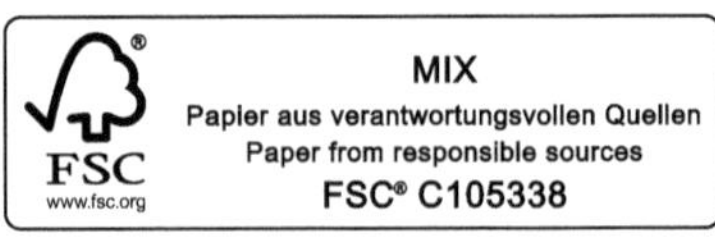

Printed by Books on Demand GmbH, Norderstedt / Germany